Scope and Standards of Practice for Registered Nurses in Care Coordination *and* Transition Management

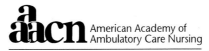

American Academy of Ambulatory Care Nursing

Many settings. Multiple roles. One unifying specialty.

American Academy of Ambulatory Care Nursing
East Holly Avenue/Box 56
Pitman, NJ 08071-0056
1-800-AMB-NURS
www.aaacn.org
aaacn@aaacn.org

Mission: Advance the art and science of ambulatory care nursing.

ISBN 978-1-940325-23-1

Publication Management by Anthony J. Jannetti, Inc.
East Holly Avenue/Box 56
Pitman, NJ 08071-0056
www.ajj.com

American Academy of Ambulatory Care Nursing (AAACN). (2016). *Scope and standards of practice for registered nurses in care coordination and transition management.* Pitman, NJ: Author.

Scope and Standards Formation Task Force

Cynthia L. Murray, BN, RN-BC (Chair)
Ambulatory Care Coordination
Southern NJ/Delaware Veterans Health System (VHA)

Shirley Burrow, MSN, RN-BC
Supervisor Population Health Care Coordination
Piedmont Healthcare, Atlanta, Georgia

Caroline M. Butt, BSN, RN
Senior Care Coordinator CCMH
Carillion Clinic, Roanoke, Virginia

Eleanor Chapital, MSN, RN-BC
Operation Enduring Freedom/Operation Iraqi
    Freedom/Operation New Dawn Program Manager
Southeast Louisiana Veterans Health System (VHA)

Dawn M. Gerz, MBA, BSN, RN, NEA-BC
Assistant Director of Ambulatory Nursing
Cleveland Clinic, Cleveland, Ohio

Mary Anne Granger, MSN, RN
Clinical Resource Leader, Care Coordination, Ambulatory
    Care Management
Maricopa Integrated Health Services, Phoenix, Arizona

Frances Gruber, MSN, RN
Patient Administrative Service Chief
South Texas Veteran Health System (VHA)

Kirsi Hayes, BSN, RN
Manager, Care Coordination – East Region
Baylor Scott & White Quality Alliance, Dallas, Texas

Lois Stauffer, MSN, RN-BC, CNL
Manager, Care Coordination
OhioHealth Physician Group, Columbus, Ohio

Advisor

Margaret F. Mastal, PhD, MSN, RN
AAACN Past President
Retired
Alexandria, Virginia

Board Liaisons

Susan M. Paschke, MSN, RN-BC, NEA-BC
AAACN Past President
Senior Director of Ambulatory Nursing
Cleveland Clinic, Cleveland Ohio

Marianne Sherman, MS, RN-BC
AAACN Past President
Retired
Denver, Colorado

Reviewers

Rabon Allen, MSN, RN
Rainbow Babies & Children's Hospital
Cleveland, Ohio

Nancy J. Birnbaum, BSN, RN-BC
Central Texas Veteran's Health System (VHA)
College Station, Texas

Mary Anne Bord-Hoffman, MN, RN-BC
San Jose Outpatient Clinic
Palo Alto California Veterans Health System (VHA)

Toyin Lawal, BSN, RN
UCLA Health
Los Angeles, California

Karen T. McKinsey, MBA, RN-BC
San Diego California Veterans Health System (VHA)

Kathy Mertens, MN, MPH, RN
UW Medicine – Harborview Medical Center
Seattle, Washington

Leslie K. Morris, BSN, RN
Texas Children's Hospital
Houston, Texas

Edtrina Moss, MSN, RN-BC, NE-BC
Michael E. DeBakey VA Medical Center (VHA)
Missouri City, Texas

Wanda C. Richards, BSN, MSM, MPA, RN
Retired United States Navy
Woodbridge, Virginia

Robbin Weaver MSN, NSII, RN
Oak Forest Health Center of Cook County Health &
    Hospital Systems
Oak Forest, Illinois

MSNCB Reviewers

Julie Alban, MSN, MPH, RN-BC
The Villages Outpatient Clinic
North Florida/South Georgia Veterans Health System
The Villages, Florida

Diane Brookes, BSN, RN, CMSRN
VA Maine HealthCare System
Augusta, Maine

Christine Chmielewski, MS, CRNP, ANP-BC, CNN-NP
Edward J. Filippone, MD, PC & Associates
Philadelphia, Pennsylvania
Center for Nursing Education and Testing
Jersey City, New Jersey

C. Westley Foster, MSN, BA, RN, CMSRN, OCN
Banner University Medical Center – Phoenix Campus
Phoenix, Arizona
Mesa Community College
Mesa, Arizona

Margery Garbin, PhD, RN
Center for Nursing Education and Testing
Jersey City, New Jersey

Darmel Hudson, BSN, RN, CCM
First Choice Health
Seattle, Washington

**Jo Ellen Inman-Puckett, MSN, MBA, RN, CNL,
    CMSRN, AHN-BC**
Carolinas HealthCare System
Charlotte, North Carolina

Angelica May, BSN, RN, CCM
Elmhurst Memorial Clinic
Elmhurst, Illinois

Table of Contents

Introduction

The American Academy of Ambulatory Care Nursing (AAACN), the specialty nursing organization for those practicing in ambulatory care settings, is responsible for establishing and maintaining the standards for ambulatory care nursing practice. To fulfill this responsibility, AAACN has published standards for professional ambulatory care nursing since 1987. The current standards include:

- 2010 – AAACN published the *Scope and Standards of Practice for Professional Ambulatory Care Nursing,* which addresses the delivery of ambulatory clinical care and administrative nursing in general.
- 2011 – AAACN published the *Scope and Standards of Practice for Professional Telehealth Nursing,* which specifically addresses professional nursing practice in the subspecialty of telehealth.

AAACN embarked on a multi-year journey developing the role of the ambulatory care registered nurse (RN) in care coordination and transition management (CCTM). The RN-CCTM Model was developed, including its dimensions, competencies, core curriculum, and online course. Additionally, AAACN included input from the Academy of Medical-Surgical Nurses (AMSN) to ensure that acute care was incorporated in this body of work that spans the continuum of care (AMSN, 2009, 2012).

This document, *Scope and Standards of Practice for Registered Nurses in Care Coordination and Transition Management,* is an evolution of AAACN's body of work and a major step forward for nurses in CCTM roles. It is the first statement of the scope and standards of practice for RNs engaged in CCTM. These roles are part of the vision of the "transformed future of health care" developed by the Committee on the Robert Wood Johnson Foundation Initiative on the Future of Nursing at the Institute of Medicine (IOM). Today's health care institutions have responded to the requirements of the Affordable Care Act (ACA) of 2010 and are in the process of changing the way health care is delivered. The ACA offers nursing multiple opportunities to facilitate health systems' improvements and the mechanics of health care delivery (IOM, 2011). CCTM roles focus on communicating and partnering with other professional health care colleagues across diverse health care settings. These settings include ambulatory care, acute care, post-acute care, long-term care facilities, and diverse community settings.

The actions and competencies within current CCTM roles have been evolving in America over the past 200 years and more intensely over the past 25 years. Yet, there has never been formal identification, specification, and/or publication of the scope and standards of practice. Doing so is a priority if nursing is to respond to the vision and challenges presented by the IOM report (2011), which includes identifying and defining nurses' contributions to health care quality, access, and value.

This publication may be used to:

1. Provide guidance for health care institutions and professional staff in regards to the organizational structure and processes (e.g., institutional policies, procedures, role descriptions and competencies) needed to facilitate RN practice in the competent provision of CCTM.
2. Guide the provision of quality nursing care during CCTM processes and activities.
3. Facilitate the development and expansion of the RN practice related to CCTM.
4. Facilitate the evaluation of the RN performance in CCTM activities (e.g., performance appraisals and peer review).
5. Stimulate participation in CCTM research and evidence-based practice.
6. Guide clinical, organizational, and health system performance improvement initiatives that optimize patient and/or population outcomes through CCTM (National Committee for Quality Assurance, 2013).
7. Guide ethical practice and patient advocacy in CCTM processes and activities.

This document is the inaugural statement of the scope and standards of practice for CCTM developed and published by AAACN. It includes:

- The historical evolution of modern day CCTM.
- The definitions of CCTM.
- The defining characteristics for the RN practicing in the CCTM role.
- An initial conceptual framework that was adapted from models cited in the care coordination and transition management core curriculum text (Haas, Swan, & Haynes, 2014). The framework offers a structure for cataloging and unifying the distinct relationships and interactions among the RN, the patient, group and/or population, the interprofessional health care team, and the resources across the health care continuum.
- Sixteen standards for the RN practicing CCTM that address both the clinical dimension and the management dimension.

This document may be used as a tool to advance professional CCTM nursing practice, patient and population health (Halpern & Boulter, 2000), and the performance outcomes of health care institutions.

Scope of Practice for Registered Nurses in Care Coordination and Transition Management (CCTM)

I. Historical Evolution of CCTM

CCTM evolved from multiple health care models that emerged in the United States dating back to the 1800s. Today's RN-CCTM Model is rooted in care management and innovative hospital and pediatric physician practices that occurred during the latter part of the 1900s. A major influence for today's model includes changes in the funding system of health care: from reimbursement on a fee-for-service basis to a capitation system (i.e., a prepaid amount of money for each patient over a specified length of time). Still other influences on today's RN-CCTM Model include the growth of health maintenance organizations (HMOs) and pilot programs of care coordination for disabled Medicaid populations. More recently, new legislation has spurred CCTM applications to new types of managed group practices serving the general population. This confluence of phenomena serves as the launch pad for the evidence-based professional model available in the *Care Coordination and Transition Management Core Curriculum* (Haas et al., 2014).

Case Management/Care Management

Case management has a long and rich history whose seeds were planted in the development of social casework in the late 1800s. It came to greater fruition in the United States in the early 1900s in the emerging disciplines of public health, nursing, and social work (Huber, 2000).

By 1990, there were two basic types of models of care management: organizational models and community-based models. The original organizational model was designed by the New England Medical Center. It is an extension of primary nursing methods and focused on the acute care hospital episode. The New England Medical Center model defined case management as a care delivery model and called it *nursing case management* (Huber, 2000). Over the years, care management has been characterized by the supervision of care or supports, monitoring the utilization patterns of high cost/high use consumers and the employment of the medical model for coordinating authorized services within a single care delivery organization (Abery, Cady, & Simunds, 2005).

The community model emanated from the Carondelet St. Mary's Community Nursing Network in Arizona. It organized bachelor- and masters-prepared nurses as care managers in a nursing HMO. They were the hub of a network of broker services that practiced beyond the acute care episode across the health care continuum. These nurses were among the first who followed the movement of high-risk clients with chronic health problems from acute care to long-term care in community settings (Huber, 2000).

However, it was the growth of HMOs in the 1990s that precipitated the widespread use of the care management approach throughout health care, insurance, and social service settings (Abery et al., 2005). The physicians and staff learned to work together, a phenomenon that is the basis of care coordination and transition management.

Growth of Health Maintenance Organizations (HMOs)

HMOs are prepaid group practices that provide both health care insurance and health care services. They date back to circa 1930 and grew slowly over the following four decades due largely to strong opposition from the medical establishment. However, they attracted enrollees because of low out-of-pocket costs and their emphasis on health promotion and illness prevention.

The enactment of the Health Maintenance Organization Act of 1973 (PL 93-222) provided major impetus for HMO growth (Social Security Administration, 1974). The Act provided funding to assist in establishing and expanding HMOs, superseding state laws that restricted the establishment of prepaid health plans, and it required employers who had over 25 employees and offered health insurance as a benefit to include an HMO option. "The purpose of the legislation was to stimulate greater competition within healthcare markets by developing outpatient alternative to expensive hospital-based treatment" (National Council on Disability, 2013, p. 1). However, in the following decade, HMOs still grew slowly due to the ongoing opposition of the medical community and HMO regulatory restrictions by individual states. But the escalation of health care costs forced the government to consider new paradigms.

In an innovative move, the government authorized Medicare payments for kidney dialysis clinics and procedures performed on an outpatient basis. This spurred the formation of physician group practices that specialized in diagnostics, surgery, rehabilitation, and other services previously performed only in hospitals. The opposition of medicine to managed care plans softened as they began to understand the financial and health benefits of managed care practices.

During the late 1980s and early 1990s, managed care plans were further credited with restricting costs. Their reputation for reducing costs through managed care practices resulted in higher enroll-ments. By 1993, they covered 51% of Americans receiving health insurance through their employer (National Council on Disability, 2013).

With general health care changing and learning new ways to manage care, the government began to focus on the soaring costs of providing health care and improving outcomes for Medicaid populations with disabilities.

Care Coordination for Populations with Disabilities

In the 1990s, Medicaid became highly concerned with the poor health outcomes and high costs of caring for children and adults with disabilities. State Medicaid agencies began to search for ways to improve care outcomes while reducing costs (Abery et al., 2005).

A combination of funds from the Centers for Medicare and Medicaid Services and private foundations established pilot programs in seven states. These pilot programs were community-based agencies made up of teams of health care professionals that coordinated the care of Medicaid recipients with disabilities. Each pilot agency developed its own model of care coordination that had unique configurations of teams of advanced nurse practitioners, registered nurses, social workers, and unlicensed personnel. All functioned under a medical director. Funding was usually allocated on a capitated basis, but some plans received additional fee-for-service funding for select benefits. Capitation granted care coordinators the option to flex the benefits (i.e., the benefits could be tailored to meet patients' individual needs) (Palsbo & Mastal, 2006).

In the pilot agencies, the teams consisted of nurses, social workers, and unlicensed personnel who coordinated care. These teams were partners with the enrollees, acting as advocates for benefits to meet each person's unique needs. They formed the communication link with physicians and other community providers, updating them regarding patients' status and outcomes. As a result, the programs were successful in reducing costs and improving the health status and quality of life of enrollees (Palsbo & Mastal, 2006). Several of the pilot agencies became very innovative and made real differences in enrollees' lives by minimizing the effects of their chronic disease and enhancing the individual's ability to improve the management of their health issues. Further, they reduced unnecessary costs and built collaborative bridges among different types of community health care professionals (Mastal, Reardon, & English, 2007).

Embracing Care Coordination: Visions for the Future

In the 21st century, health care costs continued to rise and the numbers of people without health care insurance increased. Further, technology supported the collection of data that enabled providers and payers to realize that a small percentage of persons with chronic, complex conditions consumed a high proportion of health care resources. It was obvious that chronic conditions are expensive to treat and a major driver of health care spending (Thorpe, 2013). Those who struggle with multiple illnesses combined with social complexities (e.g., mental health, substance abuse, social isolation, and homelessness) find it difficult to navigate the complex, fragmented American health care system (Craig, Eby, & Whittington, 2011).

Additionally, the Affordable Care Act of 2010 includes provisions that require individualized written "plans of care and follow up plans that move with patients longitudinally over time... Care coordination has become an innovative patient-centric interprofessional collaborative practice care delivery model that integrates the registered nurse as care coordinator and transition manager" (Haas et al., 2014, p. 3).

RNs have the knowledge and expertise to serve as the pivotal agent of the interprofessional health care team, communicating with and educating patients and caregivers, as well as all stakeholders within the system and across the continuum of care.

II. Definitions of Care Coordination and Transition Management

Although care coordination and transition management are intimately entwined, they are defined separately here to optimize understanding the meaning of each and identify how they are related.

Care Coordination Definition

"Care coordination is the deliberate organization of patient care activities between two or more participants (including the patient) involved in a patient's care to facilitate the appropriate delivery of health care services. Organizing care involves the marshalling of personnel and other resources needed to carry out all required patient care activities and is often managed by the exchange of information among participants responsible for different aspects of care" (McDonald et al., 2007; McDonald et al., 2011, p. 4).

Transition Management Definition

A critical element inherent in care coordination is transition management, which is the ongoing support of patients and their families over time as they navigate care and relationships among more than one provider and/or more than one health care setting and/or more than one health service. The need for transition management is not determined by age, time, place, or health care condition, but rather by patients' and/or families' needs for support for ongoing, longitudinal individualized plans of care and follow-up plans of care within the context of health care delivery (Haas, Swan, & Haynes, 2014, p. 3).

The processes of care coordination and transition management (Coleman & Boult, 2003, p. 556) necessitate professional assessment, patient risk identification and stratification, and identification of individual patient needs and preferences that require:

- Interprofessional collaboration and teamwork;
- Evidence-based care delivery;
- Patient and/or caregiver activation and empowerment;
- Utilization of quality and safety standards;
- Ability to work independently in the domain of nursing to identify and access community resources that meet individual, group, or population needs.

The Conceptual Basis of the RN-CCTM Model

Other models such as the Chronic Care Model (Wagner, 1998) and a Logic Model (Haas & Swan, 2014) guided the development and organization of the RN-CCTM model. The RN-CCTM model was developed as part of work by ambulatory care nurse leaders and expert panels that were sponsored by AAACN. The RN-CCTM model facilitates standardization of CCTM roles in ambulatory care as well as in acute, subacute and home health care settings. It was developed based on evidence from interprofessional literature on CCTM.

III. The Chronic Care Model as Research Guide

Initially, the Chronic Care Model (CCM) (Wagner, 1998) was used to guide AAACN's translational research project where expert panels were used to search the interprofessional literature for evidence regarding CCTM. The CCM includes the essential elements whose interactions encourage high-quality chronic disease care. "These elements include: the community; the health system; self-management support; delivery system design; decision support; and clinical information systems. Evidence-based change concepts under each element, in combination, foster productive interactions between informed patients who take an active part in their care and providers with resources and expertise" (Improving Chronic Illness Care, 2006). The CCM can be applied to a variety of health states in multiple health care settings for targeted populations. The goals are improved patient outcomes, optimal patient/provider interactive experience, and cost effectiveness. The CCM also informed the development of methods in the RN-CCTM model to use when communicating with patients, families, communities, and the interprofessional team and health agencies across the care continuum.

IV. The Logic Model as a Connection Tool

Secondly, the Logic Model served to illustrate the connections among dimensions and competencies illustrated in the RN-CCTM model and activities, interprofessional participants, and short-, medium-, and long-term outcomes (Haas et al., 2014, pp. 10-11).

AAACN initially developed and encourages the ongoing expansion of the RN-CCTM Model as the framework for RNs performing CCTM. Care coordination and transition management have long been a dimension of the professional nurse role especially in ambulatory care (Haas et al., 1995). However, CCTM activities conducted by professional nurses in ambulatory settings have often been invisible because charting or documentation in ambulatory care settings by nurses was not routinely required. Also, CCTM is within the scope of practice of other health care providers such as advanced practice registered nurses, physicians, pharmacists, and social workers.

Although other professionals also practice CCTM, it is the RN who has the knowledge and expertise to serve as the pivotal agent of the interprofessional health care team by collaborating with internal team members, leading teams, educating patients and caregivers, as well as communicating with all stakeholders within the system and across the continuum of care.

V. RN-CCTM Model

The RN-CCTM model contains two major elements for its application. First, it lists the dimensions or competencies that are essential to CCTM. These include (Haas et al., 2014, p. 9):

1. Support for self-management;
2. Advocacy;
3. Education and engagement of patient and family/caregivers;
4. Cross setting communication and transition;
5. Coaching and counseling of patients, families, and caregivers;
6. Application of the nursing process;
7. Population health management;
8. Teamwork and collaboration
9. Patient-centered care planning.

Secondly, it uses the Logic Model to link these competencies with activities, participants, and outcomes (see Figure 1).

VI. Defining Characteristics of Registered Nurses (RN) in the CCTM Role

RNs practicing in the CCTM role (adapted from AAACN, 2011; Haas et al., 2014) exhibit the following characteristics:

1. Demonstrate knowledge, skills, and attitudes requisite to the RN-CCTM dimensions.
2. Practice across the care continuum in a variety of settings, such as acute, subacute, and Patient Centered Medical Home settings such as medical offices, Accountable Care Organizations (ACOs), freestanding health clinics, nurse-managed clinics, ambulatory surgery centers, the patient's home, telehealth service environments, care coordination organizations, comprehensive health care systems, and community health care resource agencies.

Figure 1.
CCTM Depicted within a Logic Model

Situation: The Care Coordination and Transition Management (CCTM) Model evolved to standardize work of ambulatory care nurses using evidence from interdisciplinary literature on care coordination and transition management. The vision is the CCTM Model would specify dimensions of CCTM and competencies needed to perform CCTM and make possible development of knowledge, skills, and attitudes needed for each competency so the registered nurse (RN) will meet needs of patients with complex chronic illnesses (and their families) being cared for in Patient-Centered Medical Homes (PCMH), as well as traditional and nontraditional outpatient settings, and acute, subacute, and home care settings, and their preparation so work as an RN in CCTM would be recognized and reimbursed by the Centers for Medicare & Medicaid Services.

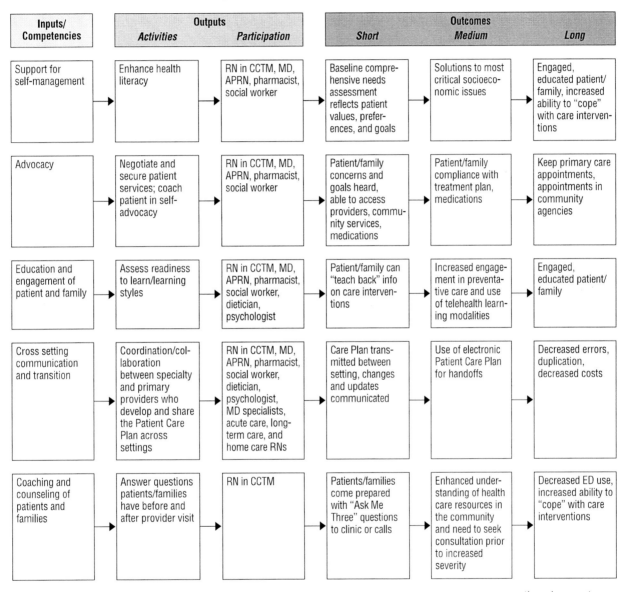

| Inputs/ Competencies | Outputs | | Outcomes | | |
	Activities	Participation	Short	Medium	Long
Support for self-management	Enhance health literacy	RN in CCTM, MD, APRN, pharmacist, social worker	Baseline comprehensive needs assessment reflects patient values, preferences, and goals	Solutions to most critical socioeconomic issues	Engaged, educated patient/ family, increased ability to "cope" with care interventions
Advocacy	Negotiate and secure patient services; coach patient in self-advocacy	RN in CCTM, MD, APRN, pharmacist, social worker	Patient/family concerns and goals heard, able to access providers, community services, medications	Patient/family compliance with treatment plan, medications	Keep primary care appointments, appointments in community agencies
Education and engagement of patient and family	Assess readiness to learn/learning styles	RN in CCTM, MD, APRN, pharmacist, social worker, dietician, psychologist	Patient/family can "teach back" info on care interventions	Increased engagement in preventative care and use of telehealth learning modalities	Engaged, educated patient/ family
Cross setting communication and transition	Coordination/collaboration between specialty and primary providers who develop and share the Patient Care Plan across settings	RN in CCTM, MD, APRN, pharmacist, social worker, dietician, psychologist, MD specialists, acute care, long-term care, and home care RNs	Care Plan transmitted between setting, changes and updates communicated	Use of electronic Patient Care Plan for handoffs	Decreased errors, duplication, decreased costs
Coaching and counseling of patients and families	Answer questions patients/families have before and after provider visit	RN in CCTM	Patients/families come prepared with "Ask Me Three" questions to clinic or calls	Enhanced understanding of health care resources in the community and need to seek consultation prior to increased severity	Decreased ED use, increased ability to "cope" with care interventions

Source: Haas, Swan, & Haynes, 2014.
© S. Haas & B.A. Swan

continued on next page

Figure 1. (continued)
CCTM Depicted within a Logic Model

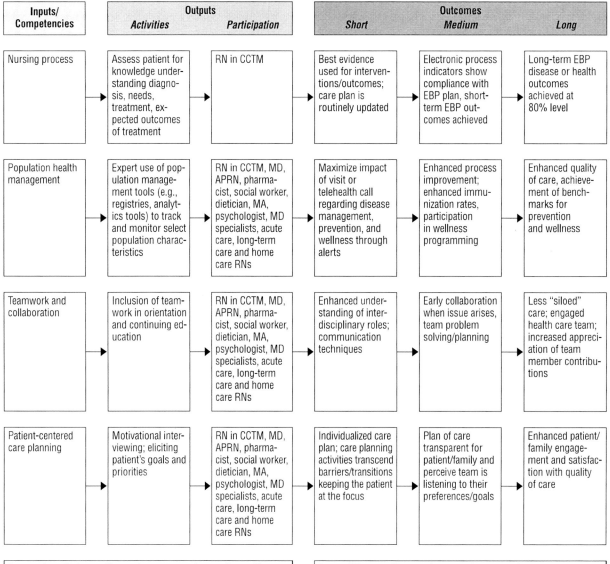

| Inputs/ Competencies | Outputs | | Outcomes | | |
	Activities	Participation	Short	Medium	Long
Nursing process	Assess patient for knowledge under-standing diagno-sis, needs, treatment, ex-pected outcomes of treatment	RN in CCTM	Best evidence used for interven-tions/outcomes; care plan is routinely updated	Electronic process indicators show compliance with EBP plan, short-term EBP out-comes achieved	Long-term EBP disease or health outcomes achieved at 80% level
Population health management	Expert use of pop-ulation manage-ment tools (e.g., registries, analyt-ics tools) to track and monitor select population charac-teristics	RN in CCTM, MD, APRN, pharma-cist, social worker, dietician, MA, psychologist, MD specialists, acute care, long-term care and home care RNs	Maximize impact of visit or telehealth call regarding disease management, prevention, and wellness through alerts	Enhanced process improvement; enhanced immu-nization rates, participation in wellness programming	Enhanced quality of care, achieve-ment of bench-marks for prevention and wellness
Teamwork and collaboration	Inclusion of team-work in orientation and continuing ed-ucation	RN in CCTM, MD, APRN, pharma-cist, social worker, dietician, MA, psychologist, MD specialists, acute care, long-term care and home care RNs	Enhanced under-standing of inter-disciplinary roles; communication techniques	Early collaboration when issue arises, team problem solving/planning	Less "siloed" care; engaged health care team; increased appreci-ation of team member contribu-tions
Patient-centered care planning	Motivational inter-viewing; eliciting patient's goals and priorities	RN in CCTM, MD, APRN, pharma-cist, social worker, dietician, MA, psychologist, MD specialists, acute care, long-term care and home care RNs	Individualized care plan; care planning activities transcend barriers/transitions keeping the patient at the focus	Plan of care transparent for patient/family and perceive team is listening to their preferences/goals	Enhanced patient/ family engage-ment and satisfac-tion with quality of care

Assumptions: Patients will use primary care settings; patients will access CCTM providers; patients will be engaged in care processes; providers will collaborate, work in teams, develop and use patient-centered care plans; organization will have EHRs that operate across settings; outcomes are shared by team, not discipline specific.

External Factors: Slow development of interdisciplinary team education and practice. Changes in reimbursement and penalties for "never events" are decreasing revenues, slow implementation of EMRs that are operable across settings, and slow development of model of care plan that moves between settings.

Source: Haas, Swan, & Haynes, 2014.
© S. Haas & B.A. Swan

3. Apply critical and analytical reasoning and astute clinical judgment (Lavery & Hughes, 2008) in order to expedite appropriate health care and treatment given that patients and/or populations often present with complex problems and/or po-tentially life-threatening conditions.

4. Provide CCTM services throughout the lifespan for individuals, families, caregivers, groups, pop-ulations, and communities.

5. Interact with patients, health care providers, and community resource agencies during face-to-face encounters or through various types of technological communication methods in order to assess and triage patient/population issues, provide nursing consultation, perform follow-up and surveillance of status and outcomes, and disseminate pertinent information to all members of the interprofessional CCTM team.

6. Apply appropriate evidence-based interventions that focus on patient safety and the quality of care:
   a) Identify and clarify the health care needs of patients/populations;
   b) Coach and counsel patients/populations;

c) Develop and maintain a written plan of care;
d) Communicate with relevant health care professionals;
e) Conduct health education;
f) Advocate for patients;
g) Coordinate appropriate health services assisting the patient to navigate the system;
h) Evaluate patient outcomes and communicate them to the health care team.

7. Partner with and advise patients, families, and caregivers in making critical health decisions, respecting their culture and values, individual needs, health goals, and treatment preferences.

8. Activate and engage with patients, families, and caregivers to optimally manage their own health care.

9. Facilitate continuity of care using interprofessional collaboration and coordination of appropriate health care services and community resources across the care continuum.

10. Serve as a clinical leader within the organization advocating for use of best evidence-based practice in implementation and evaluation of care coordination and/or transition management.

11. Design, provide, and evaluate CCTM services in accordance with relevant federal requirements, state laws, nurse practice acts, regulatory standards, and institutional policies and procedures.

12. Assume accountability for nursing services within the CCTM model, including the appropriate staff skill mix and delegation of roles and responsibilities for licensed and unlicensed nursing personnel.

13. Apply the provisions of the American Nurses Association Code of Ethics to professional CCTM practice.

14. Pursue lifelong learning that updates and expands clinical, organizational, and professional competencies, roles, and responsibilities within CCTM.

15. Identify and evaluate current research and best practices related to CCTM of populations and disseminate research findings across organizational, community, and professional arenas.

16. Take a leadership role in devising methods and implementing data analyses to identify successes and performance improvement initiatives that improve CCTM.

Standards of Practice for Registered Nurses in Care Coordination and Transition Management (CCTM)

AAACN has established these standards for CCTM nursing practice as authoritative statements that describe the responsibilities for which care coordination and/or transition management nurses are accountable. In this version, the standards have been separated into two domains: Clinical Practice and Professional Performance.

Standards of Clinical Practice

The six Clinical Practice Standards address the science and art of nursing clinical practice in CCTM through the nursing process, a rational, systematic method of planning and providing nursing care. Ida J. Orlando, one of the first nursing theorists to write about nursing process in the late 1950s, discovered common elements as she observed nurses providing patient care (Faust, 2002).

The nursing process has been refined and developed by the profession, evolving over the intervening decades. Six steps are the basis of the standards of clinical practice in nursing (ANA, 2009). These standards have built on the framework and adapted it to the CCTM practice setting.

- **Assessment:** The professional nurse systematically collects and analyzes patient(s) and/or population(s) data taking in to account the following factors: physiological, psycho-social-cultural, spiritual, economic status, developmental age, and lifestyle. The nurse identifies the presenting problem as well as the patient/population response while seeking appropriate solutions.
- **Nursing Diagnosis:** A statement that represents the nurse's clinical judgment about patient/population response to actual or potential health conditions or needs.
- **Identification of Expected Outcomes/Goals:** Actions taken by professional nurse using input from the patient/family, other health care professionals, and current scientific evidence, to identify the end objectives for patient(s) or population(s).
- **Planning:** The professional nurse outlines a set of written statements, creating an action plan that sets measureable and achievable short- and long-term goals to meet expected outcomes for patient(s) and/or population(s).
- **Implementation:** The professional nurse provides nursing care services to assist the patient(s) and/or population(s) in meeting goals through coordination of care, health promotion and ongoing health teaching, consultation with interprofessional team members, and effective documentations of all activities.
- **Evaluation:** The professional nurse's continual appraisals of the patient/population care outcomes and revising the plan of care as appropriate.

Standards of Nursing Organizational and Professional Performance

The organizational and professional performance standards identify a competent level of nursing behavior in CCTM. These behaviors include activities related to:

- Coordination of Care, Health Teaching and Health Promotion, Consultation
- Ethics
- Education
- Research and Evidence-Based Practice
- Performance Improvement
- Communication
- Leadership
- Collaboration
- Professional Practice Evaluation
- Resource Utilization
- Environment

Standard 1

Assessment

Standard

The RN practicing CCTM systematically collects comprehensive and focused data relating to health needs and concerns of a patient, group, or population as they move across the care continuum.

Competencies

CCTM nurses:

1. Collect subjective and objective information pertaining to health status from the patient, caregivers, health records, interprofessional members, and any relevant sources to coordinate care.

2. Utilize evidence-based materials related to coordination of care and health transitions to facilitate identification of appropriate interventions for improvement and maintenance of health.

3. Arrange data in a sequential manner to address anticipated or immediate needs of patients and/or populations using critical nursing judgment.

4. Synthesize data, information based on nursing knowledge with current evidence, to identify patterns and variances in continuity of health.

5. Evaluate data for anticipated patient and/or population health outcomes utilizing the nursing process.

6. Document information accurately in a legible, understandable, and accessible format.

Additional Competencies for Nurse Executives, Administrators, and Managers

CCTM nurse executives, administrators, and managers:

1. Identify specific assessment skills relevant to CCTM.

2. Utilize current evidence/practice guidelines to implement and improve data collections/decision support systems.

3. Facilitate open communications between the RN in CCTM and all entities involved in CCTM.

4. Ensure information technologies support input and retrieval of data across the care continuum.

Standard 2

Nursing Diagnoses

Standard

The RN practicing CCTM analyzes the assessment data to determine the diagnosis or issues in order to facilitate the appropriate level of care across the care continuum.

Competencies

CCTM nurses:
1. Derive a nursing diagnosis based on analysis of the assessment data and information, current nursing knowledge, and evidence-based practice.
2. State the diagnosis using standardized language and understandable, recognizable terminology.
3. Validate the diagnoses and/or issues with the patient, caregivers, interprofessional team members, and other providers when possible and where appropriate.
4. Clearly document the diagnoses and/or issues to facilitate the determination of expected outcomes and plans.
5. Prioritize diagnoses based on patient's condition, culture, age-specific needs, risk assessment, psychosocial assessment, preferences, and anticipated needs.

Additional Measurement Criteria for Nurse Executives, Administrators, and Managers

CCTM nurse executives, administrators, and managers:
1. Support staff in developing and maintaining competency in problem and/or diagnosis identification.
2. Direct education and guidance for professional nursing personnel to develop and utilize nursing problems and diagnostic statements related to CCTM.
3. Secure adequate resources for decision analysis in coordination within organizational departments and outside agencies.
4. Facilitate interprofessional collaboration in data analysis and decision(s)-making process.
5. Promote an organizational climate that supports the validation of problem and/or diagnostic statements relevant to CCTM.

Standard 3

Outcomes Identification

Standard

The RN practicing CCTM identifies expected outcomes specific to the patient, group, or population across the care continuum.

Competencies

CCTM nurses:

1. Utilize an interprofessional approach to identify goals that are realistic, specific, measurable, time-sensitive, and reportable.

2. Demonstrate the ability to incorporate patient, family, and/or caregiver in the process of identifying specific, concise, and measurable goals.

3. Prioritize goals based upon patient and family preferences and values.

4. Identify potential risks and barriers to short- and long-term goals.

5. Develop outcomes that guide care across the health care continuum.

6. Utilize a holistic, patient-centered, evidence-based approach to attaining expected outcomes.

7. Derive outcomes from assessment data and prioritized nursing diagnoses.

8. Document expected and achieved outcomes.

9. Modify expected outcomes based upon changes in the patient's status or re-evaluation of the situation.

Additional Competencies for Nurse Executives, Administrators, and Managers

CCTM nurse executives, administrators, and managers:

1. Establish and continuously improve clinical and administrative guidelines to ensure continuity of care across the care continuum.

2. Develop collaborative relationships to ensure integrated systems are available to support the delivery of patient-centered care across the continuum.

3. Support and provide resources for the identification, development, and utilization of various technologies and databases that include nursing measures and expected outcomes.

4. Facilitate the participation of the professional nurse in the monitoring and evaluation of nursing care in accordance with established professional, regulatory, and organizational standards of practice.

5. Initiate activities that improve nursing practice, organizational performance, and optimal patient and population outcomes.

Standard 4
Planning

Standard

The RN practicing CCTM develops a patient- and/or population-centered plan of care that identifies and advocates for strategies and alternatives to attain expected outcomes.

Competencies

CCTM nurses:
1. Develop a goal-oriented plan for patients and/or populations seeking care for health promotion, health maintenance, or health-related situational problems.
2. Employ current nursing knowledge and evidence-based nursing practices in the plan of care.
3. Include the patient, appropriate caregivers, and other health care professionals in shared decisions about prioritizing plans and strategies.
4. Consider patient and/or population needs in terms of age, gender, race, cultural values and practices, ethical and legal considerations, and environmental factors, as well as the anticipated risks and benefits of interventions for plan development.
5. Identify any barriers that may prevent the patient's ability to carry out the plan, such as a lack of resources or access to care.
6. Incorporate a timeline for goal-driven plan of care and achievement, reevaluation or reassessment, follow-up care, and care coordination as appropriate.
7. Assure the plan complies with organizational policies, guidelines, and evidence-based practices in the coordination and management of the care of the patient and/or population.
8. Ensure that the plan incorporates the most valid, cost-effective, evidence-based care and integrates current trends and available research.
9. Document the plan using legible, understandable, readable language and recognizable terminology.
10. Use the client's desired outcomes to plan and provide direction for other members of the CCTM team.

Additional Competencies for Nurse Executives, Administrators, and Managers

CCTM nurse executives, administrators, and managers:
1. Facilitate the development/improvement of organizational systems in which plans related to CCTM services can be developed, documented, and evaluated.
2. Promote the integration of organizational and management theories, nursing and related research findings, practice standards, and guidelines into the planning process.
3. Facilitate the development and maintenance of staff competency in planning and change processes.
4. Collaborate with appropriate departments and disciplines for the organizational system to operate more effectively and efficiently in achieving outcomes.

Standard 5

Implementation

Standard

The RN practicing CCTM implements the identified plan of care to attain expected outcomes in selected groups or individuals.

Competencies

CCTM nurses:

1. Demonstrate ability to independently implement effective, population-based nursing interventions across the health care continuum that incorporate evidence-based practice guidelines, state and regulatory agency standards, and organizational policies and procedures.

2. Prioritize interventions based on an individual or population's condition, situation, and needs along the health care continuum within organizational and regulatory requirements to attain expected outcomes.

3. Implement plans along the health continuum utilizing the unique knowledge, skills, and competencies required to track, promote, maintain, restore health, or support end-of-life situations.

4. Utilize competent, evidence-based nursing interventions during care coordination processes, with an emphasis on medical home/outpatient settings according to regulatory guidelines and organizational requirements.

5. Provide population- and age-appropriate care in a compassionate, caring, and culturally and ethnically sensitive manner.

6. Collaborate with the interprofessional health team across health care settings to effectively implement population or individual care coordination plans while maintaining privacy, fiscal accountability, and individual patient advocacy.

7. Actively acquire skills with electronic technology used to document plans, care processes, team and patient communication, and patient and organizational outcomes.

8. Utilize available technology such as electronic health records (EHRs), as well as health plans, and organizational, state, and/or regulatory electronic and other communication formats and databases to attain expected outcomes.

9. Ensure that documentation of CCTM interventions and outcomes are in the applicable records and tracking systems.

Additional Competencies for Nurse Executives, Administrators, and Managers

CCTM nurse executives, administrators, and managers:

1. Establish organizational systems that ensure implementation strategies are consistent with evidence-based practice guidelines, state and regulatory agency standards, and organizational policies and procedures.

2. Facilitate staff participation in decisions to improve population health interventions and interprofessional communication.

3. Collaborate with organizational and professional peers to improve electronic information systems and interprofessional communication formats that address health needs and improve outcomes of assigned populations of patients.

Standard 5a

Coordination of Care

Standard

The RN practicing CCTM coordinates the delivery of care within the practice setting and across health care settings.

Competencies

CCTM nurses:

1. Demonstrate accountability across the care settings in maintaining continuity of care.
2. Facilitate patient and/or population progress toward positive person-centered clinical outcomes.
3. Utilize an interprofessional approach to engage the patient, caregiver, and providers in the implementation of the plan of care across the care settings.
4. Facilitate the transition of patient/population to the appropriate level of care.
5. Educate and activate the patient and/or caregiver for optimal disease management by promoting healthy lifestyle changes in the prevention of illness across population(s).
6. Prevent disease progression by reducing risk factors.
7. Recognize and maximize opportunities to increase the quality of care.
8. Manage high-risk individuals and/or population(s) with the aim of preventing or delaying adverse outcomes.
9. Communicate relevant information to the patient, caregiver, and interprofessional health care team across the care continuum.
10. Apply effective teamwork and collaboration skills to overcome identified barriers to produce quality and effective patient outcomes.

Additional Competencies for Nurse Executives, Administrators, and Managers

CCTM nurse executives, administrators, and managers:

1. Plan the global CCTM functions that meet the population's needs and are sustainable for the health care system.
2. Establish practice standards for evidence-based care delivery.
3. Communicate and build relationships with applicable stakeholders across the care continuum.
4. Develop and validate staff competencies consistent with standards of nursing practice and organizational policies for CCTM.
5. Ensure regulatory compliance with external accrediting organization(s).

Standard 5b
Health Teaching and Health Promotion

Standard

The RN practicing CCTM employs educational strategies that promote individual, community, and population wellness.

Competencies

CCTM nurses:

1. Educate the patient and/or health care consumer about the role and benefits of CCTM as a patient-centered process across health settings.
2. Provide health teaching that addresses healthy lifestyles, risk-reducing behaviors, disease management strategies, psychosocial needs, and self-care.
3. Assess patient and/or health care consumer readiness and ability to learn, their learning need, and degree of skill and confidence for self-activation and behavioral change.
4. Use health promotion and health teaching methods appropriate to the situation and the patient and/or health care consumer's values, beliefs, health practices, developmental level, learning needs, language preference, spirituality, culture, and socioeconomic status.
5. Seek opportunities for patient and/or health care consumer feedback and evaluation of the effectiveness of teaching strategies.
6. Use information technologies to communicate health promotion and disease prevention information to the patient and/or health care consumer across the care continuum.
7. Educate patient and/or health care consumer regarding risk and benefits of proposed therapies for the intended outcomes.

Additional Competencies for Nurse Executives, Administrators, and Managers

CCTM nurse executives, administrators, and managers:

1. Synthesize empirical evidence on risk behaviors, learning theories, behavioral change theories, motivational theories, epidemiology, and other related theories and frameworks when designing health education information and programs.
2. Engage consumer alliances and advocacy groups, as appropriate, in health teaching and health promotion activities.
3. Serve as role models for healthy self-care activities and stress management.
4. Create environments that promote positive, collegial staff and patient-staff interactions.

Standard 5c
Consultation

Standard

The RN practicing CCTM as a nurse leader provides consultation to influence identified plans of care, enhance the ability of other professionals, and effect change.

Competencies

CCTM nurses:

1. Synthesize clinical data and evidence when providing consultation across the care continuum.
2. Communicate consultation recommendations to appropriate stakeholders.

Additional Competencies for Nurse Executives, Administrators, and Managers

CCTM nurse executives, administrators, and managers:

1. Facilitate the effectiveness of a consultation by involving the CCTM nurse(s), stakeholders, and members of other specialties in the decision-making process and negotiation of role responsibilities.

Standard 6

Evaluation

Standard

The RN practicing CCTM evaluates the status and progress of the patient, group, or population toward the attainment of expected outcomes and communicates the status and progress to relevant professionals across the care continuum.

Competencies

CCTM nurses:

1. Conduct systematic, ongoing, and criterion-based evaluation of the outcomes of care coordination plans in relation to facilitating clinical management across transitions of care.

2. Collaborate with the interprofessional team, patient and/or family, and community resources involved in the transitional management of care in the evaluation process.

3. Integrate current, evidence-based methods and tools in the evaluation process.

4. Use ongoing assessment strategies to revise and adapt to changes in transition management of care.

5. Assimilate and document the results of the evaluative process in easily understood language for communication to the patient and/or family, interprofessional team, and community resources.

6. Participate in a collaborative process with stakeholders to assess and assure appropriate use of interventions to facilitate care coordination and/or transition management, minimizing unnecessary treatment and patient safety risks.

7. Evaluate the effectiveness of patient care coordination plans in facilitating care across transition points.

Additional Competencies for Nurse Executives, Administrators, and Managers

CCTM nurse executives, administrators, and managers:

1. Facilitate groups of transition management professionals and other health care professionals to develop processes, systems, and tools that will enhance the analytic evaluation of outcomes.

2. Act as advocates, encouraging and empowering nursing staff and stakeholders to participate in the decision-making process related to outcome evaluation.

3. Synthesize, evaluate, and determine the impact of care coordination on the patient, family, community, and health care institution.

Standard 7
Ethics

Standard

The RN practicing CCTM applies the principles of professional nursing codes of ethics that ensure individual rights in all areas of practice.

Competencies

CCTM nurses:

1. Participate without recrimination in the identification of ethical concerns using the mechanisms provided by the applicable organization(s).
2. Contribute input and/or serve on patients' rights and ethics committees.
3. Maintain awareness of emerging ethical trends that affect patient rights.
4. Deliver nursing care that reflects the cultural, spiritual, intellectual, educational, and psychosocial differences among patients, families, or communities, and that preserves patient autonomy, dignity, and rights.
5. Advocate and support informed decisions by the patient or legally designated representative.
6. Facilitate patient rights to voice opinions regarding care and services received without recrimination, as well as their rights to have issues addressed.
7. Incorporate appropriate measures to deliver safe patient care in cases where patients are not able to act in their own best interests or do not understand the consequences of their decisions.
8. Promote access to quality health services that encompass equality, confidentiality of information, and continuity of care.

Additional Competencies for Nurse Executives, Administrators, and Managers

CCTM nurse executives, administrators, and managers:

1. Ensure written policies are in place in regard to patient rights and responsibilities, confidentiality of information, personal privacy, and self-determination.
2. Ensure information is communicated in ways that diverse populations are able to comprehend.
3. Create policies that reflect the inherent self-worth, respect, and rights that individuals have to quality health care that addresses unique physical, cultural, spiritual, and psychosocial factors.
4. Develop and update organizational policies that define process and outcome indicators related to CCTM.

Standard 8
Education

Standard

The RN practicing CCTM attains knowledge and competence that reflects current evidence-based nursing practice.

Competencies

CCTM nurses:

1. Demonstrate a commitment to lifelong learning while actively expanding their knowledge base through diverse health care setting experiences, along with organizational and health care-related educational activities.

2. Participate in continuous educational activities to expand CCTM nursing knowledge and professional issues to include the attendance of professional conferences.

3. Integrate best practice with current evidence-based research related to clinical practice, specific populations, and organizational decision-making in CCTM.

4. Identify a personal plan of knowledge expansion through self-evaluation and individual reflections that address learning and growth needs.

5. Support professional expertise by actively seeking to obtain certification in CCTM and other related professional certifications.

6. Promote professionalism by maintaining memberships in appropriate associations/organizations.

7. Seek experiences that reflect current practice to maintain knowledge, changing needs of populations, skills, abilities, and clinical practice or role performance.

8. Develop expert peer relationship networks for mentoring, coaching, and support.

9. Maintain personal/professional records that include evidence of current licensure, evaluation and validation of clinical competence, continuing education, and any certification or verification of special skill sets.

Additional Competencies for Nurse Executives, Administrators, and Managers

CCTM nurse executives, administrators, and managers:

1. Maintain a learning environment that encourages and supports the staff in advancing knowledge, clinical practice, and organizational performance using evidence-based practices.

2. Promote programs that encourage or reward achievement of educational excellence through attainment of professional certifications in nursing specialties or related programs.

3. Provide access to education and learning opportunities to promote clinical competence and professional development as a shared responsibility of the organization and the professional nursing staff.

4. Establish a work environment conducive to sharing educational findings, experiences, and ideas.

Standard 9
Research and Evidence-Based Practice

Standard

The RN practicing CCTM integrates relevant research findings into practice in order to optimize standards of care and best practice for diverse individuals/populations, to promote continuous improvement, and to advance the profession.

Competencies

CCTM nurses:
1. Review and evaluate current research and best practices relevant to the CCTM of populations.
2. Utilize interventions substantiated by evidence-based practice or research.
3. Participate in research activities – including those that must be approved by an institutional review board (IRB) – related to CCTM of populations within the guidelines of the individual facility, national statutes, and regulations.
4. Identify population health concerns suitable for CCTM research.
5. Disseminate relevant nursing research findings in CCTM across organizational, community, and professional forums.

Additional Competencies for Nurse Executives, Administrators, and Managers

CCTM nurse executives, administrators, and managers:
1. Use research findings and/or evidence-based practices in the development of all applicable policies, procedures, and guidelines.
2. Critique research for application to CCTM settings and practice.
3. Ensure that research conducted in the clinical and/or organizational environment undergoes review and approval by an IRB and adheres to ethical principles.
4. Encourage an environment of continuous improvement by promoting clinical investigation and best practices.
5. Ensure that organizational resources are adequately allocated and deployed so that nurses update their knowledge base through educational activities, engage in evidence-based nursing practice, participate in quality of care and improvement initiatives, and use nursing, clinical, and health system research findings.
6. Balance the cost and benefits to staff, patients, and the organization when participating in research studies.

Standard 10

Performance Improvement

Standard

The RN practicing CCTM enhances the quality and effectiveness of professional practice, organizational systems, and population health outcomes.

Competencies

CCTM nurses:

1. Continuously monitor CCTM nursing practice to identify opportunities for improving safety, quality of care, and health outcomes.
2. Implement the nursing process in a responsible, accountable, and ethical manner.
3. Identify opportunities for improvement that will enhance patients' experience and promote population health.
4. Participate in the tracking, recording, analysis, and synthesis of data to improve CCTM across the care continuum.
5. Identify barriers to care across services and organizations.
6. Participate in and/or lead interprofessional teams on system redesign projects aimed at improving CCTM across different services and facilities.
7. Integrate data analysis and performance improvement initiatives into practice with the aim of improving CCTM, patient outcomes, organizational effectiveness, and efficiency.
8. Obtain and maintain professional certification in the area of CCTM.

Additional Competencies for Nurse Executives, Administrators, and Managers

CCTM nurse executives, administrators, and managers:

1. Plan, direct, and evaluate CCTM nursing services as it applies to data, documentation, interprofessional interactions, and cross-system delivery of care.
2. Provide leadership to direct the design, implementation, and evaluation of nursing practice within a CCTM framework.
3. Engage in initiatives that identify and define nurse-sensitive indicators.
4. Implement organizational policies and procedures specific to the practice of CCTM consistent with applicable federal and state statutes, rules, regulations, and accepted standards of nursing practice.
5. Obtain and maintain professional certification in the area of CCTM.
6. Foster communication, collaboration, and coordination of improvement efforts across the health care continuum.
7. Lead quality of care and performance improvement initiatives and delegate activities as appropriate.

Standard 11
Communication

Standard

The RN practicing CCTM communicates effectively using a variety of formats, tools, and technologies to build professional relationships and deliver care across the continuum.

Competencies

CCTM nurses:

1. Promote active communication using a method or manner that enhances learning and the sharing of information.
2. Evaluate personal skills and styles of communication to identify areas needing improvement and/or education.
3. Share best practices with peers, requesting feedback and evaluation.
4. Maintain professional communication(s) with members of the health care team, families, and stakeholders to promote effective interactions.
5. Create a positive environment that fosters an attitude of information sharing and learning.
6. Share with the health care team hazards or barriers that could have a negative effect on patients and/or caregivers.
7. Seek opportunities to create positive mentoring relationships in regard to CCTM, as well as individual and departmental practices.
8. Share and communicate knowledge and skills obtained from professional conferences and seminars to CCTM colleagues and staff.
9. Exemplify an engaged attitude and professional nursing practice that fosters a sense of excellence and enthusiasm among peers and colleagues.

Additional Competencies for Nurse Executives, Administrators, and Managers

CCTM nurse executives, administrators, and managers:

1. Create a positive environment of collegiality and trust through shared professional communication, experiences, and decision-making among new and experienced CCTM staff.
2. Seek, evaluate, and implement communication tools and technologies that improve CCTM.
3. Act as a resource to and serve as an example of positive, professional communication with all members of the interprofessional health care team.
4. Recognize individual or group accomplishments to foster a sense of professional pride and intradepartmental expertise.
5. Engage with professional and organizational decision-making bodies to improve care practices, environment, and patient or population outcomes.

Standard 12
Leadership

Standard

The RN practicing CCTM acquires and utilizes leadership behaviors in practice settings, within the profession, and across the care continuum.

Competencies

CCTM nurses:

1. Demonstrate respect for human dignity and worth by valuing people as the central asset of the work setting, the profession, and the community.
2. Assume an active role as a team player and team builder to create and maintain healthy, safe work environments in practice and community settings.
3. Demonstrate a commitment to continuous ongoing education for self and others.
4. Serve as a mentor for new staff, colleagues, and students by identifying and engaging in learning opportunities.
5. Provide oversight of licensed and unlicensed assistive personnel in assigned or delegated tasks consistent with their defined roles, nursing practice regulations, and professional standards.
6. Initiate and/or participate in continuous quality health and improvement activities as a means to advance individual, community, and population wellness.
7. Lead and actively participate in projects, community education, committees, and councils by serving in key roles in the practice and community settings.
8. Collaborate with colleagues, supervisors, and co-workers to build and maintain effective, dynamic, and interprofessional teams.
9. Establish an environment of trust, collaboration, and continuous learning by applying critical thinking skills to understand and learn from shared and individual experiences.
10. Promote the advancement and strength of the nursing profession through active membership and leadership in professional and community organizations.

Additional Competencies for Nurse Executives, Administrators, and Managers

CCTM nurse executives, administrators, and managers:

1. Define a clear vision for CCTM by identifying shared goals.
2. Develop plans to implement and measure CCTM practices, organizational performance, care improvements, and outcomes.
3. Create a collegial, shared decision-making environment that incorporates organizational culture, values, and perspectives.
4. Identify the need for change and promote improvements in a collaborative manner using evidence-based guidelines and practices.
5. Utilize the power of positive influence with decision-making bodies to resolve conflict and formulate policy.
6. Lead initiatives that enhance CCTM practice, expand health system capabilities, and improve the health of individuals as well as the community.
7. Serve as a model of authentic and engaged leadership, inspiring shared practice and future vision development within CCTM.
8. Champion an environment conducive to innovation, communication, and positive changes based on evidence, research, advances in the health care industry, and organization strategic and financial directions.
9. Represent CCTM nursing on appropriate decision-making boards and committees of the organization to provide input on program planning and system changes that impact CCTM and patient care outcomes.

Standard 13

Collaboration

Standard

The RN practicing CCTM interacts with the patient, family members, caregivers, and health care professionals to foster professional relationships that improve population health.

Competencies

CCTM nurses:

1. Apply critical-thinking skills and use appropriate clinical judgments when implementing population health interventions or planning effective care for groups or individual patients and their families.
2. Partner with interprofessional team members in diverse settings regarding the promotion, prevention, and restoration of health in populations.
3. Recognize that populations are composed of individual patients.
4. Provide outreach to patients and their caregivers to identify health or psychosocial issues used in the development of an appropriate plan of care.
5. Coordinate with local and community resources to improve the health of populations or individual patients.
6. Communicate recommended intervention(s) and plan(s) of care with expected outcomes with individual patients or caregivers and applicable members of the interprofessional team.
7. Interface with peers using shared decision-making to implement practice(s) to improve population health and CCTM performance and standards.

Additional Competencies for Nurse Executives, Administrators, and Managers

CCTM nurse executives, administrators, and managers:

1. Represent CCTM through collaboration on appropriate decision-making boards and committees within the organization and the community.
2. Support nurses practicing in CCTM roles by identifying issues and celebrating successes.
3. Provide and promote education and resources to support the practice of CCTM within the organization.
4. Serve as a resource to keep the CCTM team current with organizational practices, policies, procedures, and national guidelines for population care.
5. Partner with the interprofessional team in the development of evidence-based CCTM practices.

Standard 14
Professional Practice Evaluation

Standard

The RN practicing CCTM evaluates his or her own nursing practice in relation to patient outcomes, organizational policies, procedures, job descriptions, nursing professional standards, and relevant governmental regulations and statutes.

Competencies

CCTM nurses:

1. Utilize an ongoing and systematic evaluation of work processes and personal performance.
2. Create a plan utilizing patient data that evaluates ongoing effectiveness of interventions.
3. Provide documentation of interventions that includes evaluation of related outcomes.
4. Participate in self-reflective and self-evaluative activities to improve clinical practice.
5. Engage in organizational performance reviews on a regular basis to identify strengths and opportunities for growth, as well as to set performance goals/objectives for the future.
6. Utilize the organization's systems and tools to perform timely reviews of CCTM practice(s).
7. Exhibit competence of work performance through regular review, verification of credentials, participation in ongoing education, and updates of procedures, equipment, and regulatory guidelines.
8. Participate in department and organizational peer mentoring, coaching, and peer review as appropriate.

Additional Competencies for Nurse Executives, Administrators, and Managers

CCTM nurse executives, administrators, and managers:

1. Establish a culture of excellence within the organization through thoughtful, consistent review and evaluation of evidence-based practices and quality measures.
2. Institute a process of employee performance appraisal that may encompass management feedback, peer reviews, patient and/or family comments, and physician responses.
3. Support and facilitate staff involvement in the identification of clinical, ethical, and legal issues through participation in risk management and peer review.
4. Develop standardized tools and coaching procedures for staff skills to assess, evaluate, and improve performance.

Standard 15

Resource Utilization

Standard

The RN practicing CCTM utilizes appropriate resources to plan and facilitate services that are safe, effective, and fiscally responsible.

Competencies

CCTM nurses:

1. Partner with patients and caregivers to assess individual health care needs and target the resources available to achieve desired outcomes, and assist with access to necessary resources.
2. Utilize appropriate resources to improve population health outcomes.
3. Evaluate resources for potential for harm, complexity of the task, cost effectiveness, and desired outcome when considering resource allocation.
4. Delegate care to appropriate health care workers when RN level of care is not appropriate, following applicable laws and policies.
5. Identify evidence-based practices when evaluating resource allocation.
6. Modify CCTM practice when necessary to promote optimal interaction between health care consumers, care providers, and the usage of technology.
7. Educate and support patients and caregivers to become informed consumers about the options, costs, risks, and benefits of health care services.

Additional Competencies for Nurse Executives, Administrators, and Managers

CCTM nurse executives, administrators, and managers:

1. When allocating resources, evaluate the availability, potential for harm, effectiveness, efficiency, cost, benefits, and the impact on CCTM program and organization.
2. Advocate for resources to include technology that enhances CCTM interventions and outcomes and improves organizational performance.
3. Ensure that written organizational charts delineate nursing authority, accountability, and lines of communication among nurses and other members of the interprofessional team.
4. Provide clearly defined, written descriptions and performance standards for nursing assistive personnel, outlining the accountability within the scope of practice and their role within the interprofessional team.
5. Plan staffing within organizational guidelines to ensure that sufficient nurses and nursing assistive personnel are available to deliver high quality CCTM in a safe manner.
6. Evaluate economic factors when choosing innovative CCTM solutions that result in safe, accessible, effective, and efficient practices.

Standard 16

Environment

Standard

The RN practicing CCTM actively engages in organizational initiatives that create and maintain an environment that is safe, hazard-free, ergonomically correct, confidential, and comfortable for patients, visitors, and staff.

Competencies

CCTM nurses:

1. Participate in orientation and education programs that identify and evaluate current processes and best practices that enhance the creation and maintenance of a safe, hazard-free, confidential, ergonomically correct, and comfortable work/patient care setting.
2. Monitor and identify the status and the quality of the environment of care.
3. Make recommendations to ensure that the environment is accessible, safe, and functional for patients, staff, and visitors.
4. Utilize preventive and screening programs and appropriate interventions if untoward occupational exposure occurs and/or if risk to occupational exposure is reasonably anticipated.
5. Maintain confidentiality of employee exposure to untoward exposure, treatment, and follow-up.
6. Comply with organizational policies, protocols, guidelines, and evidence-based practices addressing the prevention of infection, allergic reactions, disposal of bio hazardous waste, and maintenance of a safe and comfortable environment.
7. Maintain the physical space and professional practices that ensure patients have access to care, ensuring privacy, security, and confidentiality of personal information.
8. Utilize up-to-date medications, equipment, supplies, and technology in the practice environment.
9. Ensure that the care environment accommodates the delivery of CCTM practices and addresses age-specific, disability-specific, and diverse population needs.

Additional Competencies for Nurse Executives, Administrators, and Managers

CCTM nurse executives, administrators, and managers:

1. Utilize applicable federal and state rules regulations, organizational policies, and evidence-based practice to determine the level of resources needed for safe, quality patient care.
2. Implement policies and procedures that address training in the use of personal protective equipment, while monitoring, documenting, and reporting adverse events.
3. Implement written policies and procedures regarding confidentiality, infection control, fire and safety, security, harassment, equipment management, hazardous waste handling, and emergency situations.
4. Ensure a private and secure environment that maintains the confidentiality of patient information, and considers the following:
   a. Access to and security of computer resources.
   b. Sound transmission and issues of privacy and confidentiality.
   c. Security and safety with each patient encounter.
5. Ensure the remote environment of care meets industry standards of confidentiality, safety, security, and ergonomics.
   a. Lighting, space, temperature, and environmental services.
   b. Accessibility of resources, references, and personal break facilities.
   c. Accessibility and functionality of an environment for staff, patients, and visitors with disabilities.
6. Provide an organizational chart that delineates nursing authority, accountability, and lines of communication among the members of the CCTM health care team.

Standard 16

Environment (continued)

7. Ensure compliance with federal, state, territory, or commonwealth statues, rules, regulations, and accepted standards of evidence-based nursing practice by providing written position descriptions that define and specify responsibilities and performance requirements of CCTM staff.

8. Document and report participation in educational safety programs by interprofessional team members.

9. Implement current standards of practice and clinical guidelines to ensure the provision of care across the care continuum.

10. Maintain employee records that include evidence of current licensure, evaluation and validation of clinical competence, continuing education, certification, and any specialty skill(s).

Glossary

Many terms in nursing and health care have multiple meanings and can be used in multiple contexts. Certain terms are defined to clarify the intent and application of these standards. Terms not defined are assumed either to have a generally acceptable meaning and interpretation, or to require contextual interpretation depending on the setting and application.

Adverse Event – Unnecessary patient injury, harm, pain, suffering, or death resulting from health care management.

Advocacy – Act or process of championing support on behalf of another.

Algorithm – A step-by-step procedure that is explicit and in logical order to achieve a specific result.

Assessment – A systemic, dynamic process by which the registered nurse – through interaction with the patient, family, groups, communities, populations, and health care providers – collects and organizes data. Assessment may include the following dimensions: physical, psychological, socio-cultural, spiritual, cognitive, functional abilities, developmental, economic, and lifestyle.

Care Coordination – The deliberate organization of patient care activities between two or more participants (including the patient) involved in a patient's care to facilitate the appropriate delivery of health care services. Organizing care involves the marshaling of personnel and other resources needed to carry out all required patient care activities and is often managed by the exchange of information among participants responsible for different aspects of care.

Care Transitions – A change in the level of service or location of providers of care as patients move within the health system.

Caregiver – Individual (e.g., a family member, friend, or companion) over the age of 18 who provides care and/or support.

Certification – Process that uses predetermined standards to validate and recognize an individual's knowledge, skills, and abilities in a defined functional and clinical area of specialty practice approved by the American Board of Nursing Specialties (ABNS) as an area of specialty practice.

Clinical Practice Guidelines – Statements that have been systematically developed based on evidence to assist practitioners and patients in making decisions about appropriate health care for specific clinical circumstances.

Collaboration – Working together toward a common goal; to pursue a common purpose and a sharing of knowledge to resolve problems, decide issues, and set goals within a structure of collegiality.

Competence – Having the ability to demonstrate the knowledge, technical, critical thinking, and interpersonal skills necessary to perform one's job responsibilities.

Competency – An expected level of performance that integrates knowledge, skills, abilities, and judgment.

Confidentiality – To protect the patient's and family's right to privacy regarding information the nurse or institution holds about the patient.

Continuity of Care – Health care that remains consistent and uninterrupted throughout the care process.

Continuum of Care (Care Continuum) – Over the course of the patient's life, the patient will receive health-related care from a variety of health care and service professionals in a variety of health care settings.

Critical Thinking – A deliberate, nonlinear process of collecting, interpreting, analyzing, drawing conclusions about presenting, and evaluating information that is both factual and belief-based. This is demonstrated in nursing by clinical judgment, which includes ethical, diagnostic, and therapeutic dimensions and research.

Education Process – Systematic planned course of action consisting of two major interdependent operations: teaching and learning.

Electronic Health Record – A secure, real-time, point-of-care, patient-centric information resource for clinicians.

Engagement in Health Care – Actions individuals must take to obtain the greatest benefit from the health care services available to them.

Environment – A complex interrelationship of factors external to the organization as well as those within the health care organization by which the patient/population is surrounded, which affects care delivery services.

Ergonomics – The scientific discipline concerned with the interactions between humans and other elements of a system, and the profession that applies theory, principles, data, and methods to system design in order to optimize human wellbeing and overall system performance.

Ethics – A philosophical framework for examining values as they relate to human behaviors; how behaviors are viewed as right or wrong, good or bad, concerned with both the motives and the outcomes of actions.

Evidence-Based Practice – The conscientious, explicit, and judicious use of current best evidence in making decisions about the care of individual patient; combines research and clinical expertise.

Expected Outcomes – Anticipated results of a health care process that are measurable, desirable, and translate into observable behaviors.

Family – Family members are defined by the patient in his or her own terms and may include individuals related by blood, marriage, or in self-defined relationships. (This definition is intended to include the family in nursing care as appropriate. It is not intended as a legal definition of family.)

Hazardous Conditions – Any set of circumstances (exclusive of the disease, disorder, or condition for which the patient is undergoing care, treatment, and services) defined by the organization that significantly increases the likelihood of a serious adverse outcome.

Health Care Team – Includes the patient, family, and other members of the health care system who are involved in the development and implementation of the care plan.

Informatics – Use and support the use of information and technology to communicate, manage knowledge, mitigate error, and support decision-making.

Interprofessional Team – A group of individuals from different disciplines working and communicating with each other, providing his/her knowledge, skills, and attitudes to augment and support the contributions of others.

Leader – The person who provides guidance, direction, and/or oversight responsibilities for CCTM.

Nurse-Sensitive Indicator – Structures of care and care processes related to nursing practice that link to care outcomes.

Nursing – The protection, promotion, and optimization of health and abilities; prevention of illness and injury; alleviation of suffering through the diagnosis and treatment of human response; and advocacy in the care of individuals, families, communities, and populations.

Nursing Code of Ethics – A guide for carrying out nursing responsibilities in a manner consistent with quality in nursing care; and expression of nursing's own understanding of its commitment to society; the ethical obligations and duties of every individual who enters the nursing profession.

Nursing Informatics – A specialty that integrates nursing science, computer science, and information science to manage and communicate data, information, and knowledge in nursing practice.

Nursing Process – The essential core of practice for the RN to deliver holistic, patient-focused care.

Organization – Used interchangeably with *setting*. A broad term to describe the practice setting. This may be a physician office, medical center, hospital, managed care facility, pharmaceutical company, or health care system.

Orientation – A structured plan created by the organization to "on-board" new staff to provide smooth assimilation into a new position; key components include a general organizational overview, department specifics, and individualized job duties.

Outcomes Measurement – The collection and analysis of data using predetermined outcomes indicators for the purposes of making decisions about health care.

Patient – Recipient of nursing practice. The term *patient* is used to provide consistency and brevity, bearing in mind that other terms such as *client, individual, resident, family, groups, communities,* or *populations* might be better choices in some instances. When the patient is an individual, the focus is on the health state, problems, or needs of the individual. When the patient is a family or group, the focus is on the health state of the unit as a whole or the reciprocal effects of the individual's health state on others. When the patient is a community or population, the focus is on personal and environmental health and the health risk(s) of the community or population.

Patient Advocacy – The support and empowerment of patients to make informed decisions, navigate the health care system to access appropriate care, and build strong partnerships with providers, while working toward system improvement and patient-centered care.

Patient Education – (1) The process of influencing patient behavior and producing the changes in knowledge, skills, and attitudes necessary to maintain or improve health. (2) A process of assisting people to learn health-related behaviors that they can incorporate into everyday life with the goal of optimal health and independence.

Performance Improvement – Systematic analysis of the structure, processes, and outcomes within systems for the purpose of improving the delivery of care.

Plan of Care – A written set of actions developed by the interprofessional team, outlining the care to be provided to an individual/family/population to resolve/support health care issues identified through assessment. It guides in the ongoing provision of care and assists in the evaluation of that care.

Population – All persons in a defined subgroup with specific characteristics, such as a diagnosis, age group or claims history.

Population Health – Encompasses the ability to assess the health needs of a specific population; implement and evaluate interventions to improve the health of that population; and provide care for individual patient(s) in the context of the culture, health status, and health needs of the population(s) of which that patient is a member.

Quality Improvement – A systematic and continuous action leading to measurable improvement in health care services and/or the health status of targeted patient groups.

Risk Stratification – Proactively identify and outreach to at-risk patients to develop patient-centered care planning.

Safe – Avoiding injuries to patient(s) and/or population(s) from the care that is intended to help them.

Self-Care – Patients learn to care for themselves and participate in collaborative goal-setting and decision-making.

Self-Efficacy – A person's confidence in his/her ability to carry out behaviors necessary to achieve the desired goal.

Standard – An authoritative statement developed and disseminated by a professional organization or governmental or regulatory agency by which the quality of practice, services, research, or education can be judged.

State Practice Acts – A combination of laws and regulations that define and regulate the practice of medicine, nursing, and other health professions.

Teamwork and Collaboration – Effectively functioning within nursing and interprofessional teams, fostering open communication, mutual respect, and shared decision-making to achieve quality patient care.

Teamwork in Health Care – A dynamic process involving two or more health professionals with complementary backgrounds and skills, sharing common health goals, and exercising concerted physical and mental effort in assessing, planning, or evaluating patient care.

Transition Management in the Context of Practice of the RN – The ongoing support of patients and their families over time as they navigate care and relationships among more than one provider and/or more than one health care setting and/or more than one health care service. The need for transition management is not determined by age, time, place, or health care condition, but rather by patients' and/or families' needs for support for ongoing, longitudinal, individualized plans of care and follow-up plans of care within the context of health care delivery.

Transitional Care – (1) A set of actions designed to ensure the coordination and continuity of health care as patients transfer between different locations or different levels of care within the same location. Representative locations include (but are not limited to): hospitals, sub-acute and post-acute nursing facilities, the patient's home, primary and specialty care offices, and long-term care facilities. (2) A broad range of time-limited services designed to ensure health care continuity, avoid preventable poor outcomes among at-risk populations, and promote the safe and timely transfer of patients from one level of care to another or from one type of setting to another.

References

Abery, B., Cady, R., & Simunds, E. (2005). Health care coordination for persons of disabilities: Its meaning and importance. *Impact, 18*(1), 8-9. Retrieved from http://ici.umn.edu/products/impact/181/default.html

Academy of Medical-Surgical Nurses (AMSN). (2009). *Core curriculum for medical-surgical nursing* (4th ed.). Pitman, NJ: Author.

Academy of Medical-Surgical Nurses (AMSN). (2012). *Scope and standards of medical-surgical nursing practice* (5th ed.). Pitman, NJ: Author.

American Academy of Ambulatory Care Nursing (AAACN). (2010). *Scope and standards of practice for professional ambulatory care nursing* (8th ed.). Pitman, NJ: Author.

American Academy of Ambulatory Care Nursing (AAACN). (2011). *Scope and standards of practice for professional telehealth nursing* (5th ed.). Pitman, NJ: Author.

American Nurses Association (ANA). (2009). Nursing: A common thread amongst all nurses. *Nursing's Social Policy Statement* (2nd ed.). Silver Spring, MD: Author.

American Nurses Association (ANA). (2010). *Scope and standards of practice: Nursing*. Silver Spring, MD: Author.

American Nurses Association (ANA). (2012). *Care coordination and registered nurses' essential role position statement*. Silver Spring, MD: ANA Congress on Nursing Practice and Economics, ANA Board of Directors.

American Nurses Association (ANA). (2015). *Code of ethics for nurses with interpretative statements*. Silver Spring, MD: Author.

Care Continuum Alliance. (2012). *Implementation and evaluation: A population health guide for primary care models*. Washington, DC: Author.

Coleman, E., & Boult, C. (2003). Improving the quality of transitional care for persons with complex care needs. *Journal of the American Geriatrics Society, 51*(4), 556-557.

Craig, D., Eby, D., & Whittington, J. (2011). *Care coordination model: Better care at lower costs for people with multiple health and social needs*. IHI Innovation Series white paper. Cambridge, MA: Institute for Healthcare Improvement. Retrieved from http://www.ihi.org/resources/pages/IHIWhitePapers/IHICareCoordinationModelWhitePaper.aspx

Faust, C. (2002). Orlando's deliberate nursing process: A practice application in an extended care facility. *Journal of Gerontological Nursing, 28*(7), 8-14.

Haas, S.A., & Swan, B.A. (2014). Developing the value proposition for the role of the registered nurse in care coordination and transition management in ambulatory care settings. *Nursing Economic$, 31*(2), 70-79.

Haas, S.A., Swan, B.A., & Haynes, T.S. (Eds.) (2014). *Care coordination and transition management core curriculum*. Pitman, NJ: American Academy of Ambulatory Care Nurses.

Halpern, R., & Boulter, P. (2000). *Population-based healthcare: Definitions and applications*. Boston: Tufts Managed Care Institute.

Huber, D.L. (2000). The diversity of case management models. *Lippincott's Case Management, 5*(6), 248-255.

Improving Chronic Illness Care (ICIC). (2006). *The Chronic Care Model: Model elements*. Retrieved from http://www.improvingchroniccare.org/index.php?p=Model_Elements&s=18

Institute for Health and Technology Transformation. (2012). *Population health management: A roadmap for provider-based automation in a new era of healthcare*. Retrieved from http://ihealthtran.com/pdf/PHMReport.pdf

Institute of Medicine (IOM). (2011). *The future of nursing: Leading change, advancing health*. Washington, DC: The National Academies Press.

Jessie, A.T., Johnson, S.A., & Trehearne, B.E. (2014). Population health management. In S.A. Hass, B.A. Swan, & T.S. Haynes (Eds.), *Care coordination and transition management core curriculum*. Pitman, NJ: American Academy of Ambulatory Care Nurses.

Jones, D.S., Hoffmann, L., & Quinn, S. (2009). *21st century medicine: A new model for medical education and practice*. Retrieved from http://www.marthaherbert.org/library/IFM-White-paper-21stCenturyMedicine.pdf

Kim, C.S., & Flanders, S.A. (2013). In the clinic: Transitions of care. *Annals of Internal Medicine, 158*(5 Pt 1), ITC3-1.

Lavery, J., & Hughes, W. (2008). *Critical thinking: An introduction to the basic skills* (5th ed.). Ontario, Canada: Broadview Press.

Mastal, M.F., Reardon, M.E., & English, M. (2007). Innovations in disability care coordination organizations. *Professional Case Management, 12*(1), 27-36.

McDonald, K., Schultz, E.S., Albin, L., Pineda, N., Lonhart, J., Sundaram, V., & Malcolm, E. (2011). *Care coordination measures atlas* (AHRQ Publication No. 11-0023-EF). Rockville, MD: Agency for Healthcare Research and Quality.

McDonald, K., Sundaram, V. Bravada, D., Lewis, R., Lin, N., Kraft, S.A., & Owens, D.K. (2007). Care coordination. In K. Shojania, K. McDonald, R. Wachter, & D. Owens (Eds.), *Closing the quality gap: A critical analysis of quality improvement strategies* (AHRQ Publication No. 04 (07)-0051-7). Technical Review 9 (Prepared by Stanford UCSF Evidence-Based Practice Center under contract No. 290-02-0017). Vol. 7. Rockville, MD: Agency for Healthcare Research and Quality.

National Committee for Quality Assurance (NCQA). (2013). *Standards and guidelines for the accreditation and certification of disease management programs*. Washington, DC: Author.

National Council on Disability. (2013). *Appendix B: A brief history of managed care*. Retrieved from http://www.ncd.gov/policy/appendix-b-brief-history-managed-care

Palsbo, S., & Mastal, M. (2006). *Disability care coordination organizations: The experience of Medicaid managed care programs for people with disabilities*. Retrieved from http://www.chcs.org/resource/disability-care-coordination-organizations-the-experience-of-medicaid-managed-care-programs-for-people-with-disabilities/

Social Security Administration. (1974). *Health Maintenance Organization Act of 1973*. Retrieved from http://www.ssa.gov/policy/docs/ssb/v37n3/v37n3p35.pdf

Thorpe, K. (2013). Treated disease prevalence and spending per treated case drove most of the growth in health care spending in 1987-2009. *Health Affairs, 32*(5), 851-858.

Von Korff, M., Gruman, J., Schaefer, J., Curry, S.J., & Wagner, E.H. (1997). Collaborative management of chronic illness. *Annals of Internal Medicine, 127*(12), 1097-1102.

Wagner, E.H. (1998). Chronic disease management: What will it take to improve care for chronic illness? *Effective Clinical Practice, 1*(1), 2-4. Retrieved from http://ecp.acponline.org/augsep98/cdm.htm

Additional Readings

Anderson, S., Marrie, J., Vande, J., & Hanratty, R. (2013). Implementation of a clinical pharmacy specialist (CPS)-managed telephonic hospital discharge follow-up program in a patient-centered medical home. *Population Health Management, 16*(4), 235-241.

Camicia, M., Chamberlain, B., Finnie, R.R., Nalle, M., Lindeke, L.L., Lorenz, L., ... McMenamin, P. (2012). The value of nursing care coordination: A white paper of the American Nurses Association. *Nurse Outlook, 61*(6), 490-501.

Ciprano, P.F., Bowles, B., Dailey, M., Dykes, P., Lamb, G., & Naylor, M. (2013). The importance of health information technology in care coordination and transitional care. *Nursing Outlook, 61*(6), 475-489.

Daughtridge, G.W., Archibald, T., & Conway, P.H. (2014). Quality improvement of care transitions and the trend of composite hospital care. *JAMA American Medical Association 311*(10) 1013-1014.

Goldman, B., & Mastal, M.F. (2005). Coordinated care for children in DC: Health Services for Children with Special Needs, Inc. *Impact, 18*(1), 18-19. Retrieved from http://ici.umn.edu/products/impact/181/default.html

Greysen, S.R., Hoi-Cheung, D., Garcia, V., Kessel, E., Sarkar, U., Goldman, L., ... & Kushel, M. (2014). "Missing pieces" – Functional, social & environmental barriers to recovery for vulnerable older adults transitioning from hospital to home. *The American Geriatrics Society, 62*(8), 1556-1561.

Hewner, S. (2014). A population-based care transition model for chronically ill elders. *Nursing Economic$, 32*(3), 109-117.

Hughes, R.G. (Ed.). (2008). *Patient safety and quality: An evidence-based handbook for nurses.* Rockville, MD: Agency for Healthcare Research and Quality. Retrieved from http://www.rwjf.org/content/dam/web-assets/2008/04/patient-safety-and-quality

Jacquin, L. (2014). A strategic approach to healthcare transformation. *Healthcare Financial Management, 68*(4), 73-80.

Jing, L., Young, R., & Williams, M.V. (2014). Optimizing transitions of care to reduce hospitalizations. *Cleveland Clinic Journal of Medicine* Volume, 81(5), 312-320.

Jones, M., & Smith, P. (2013). Population-focused nursing: Advocacy for vulnerable populations in an RN-BSN program. *Public Health Nursing, 31*(5), 463-471.

Korff, M.V., Gruman, J., Schaefer, J., Curry, S.J., & Wagner, E.H. (1997, December 15). Collaborative management of chronic illness. *Annals of Internal Medicine, 127*(12), 1097-1102.

Kurtzman, E., & Dailey, M. (2013). *Framework for measuring nurses' contributions to care coordination.* Retrieved from http://www.nursingworld.org/Framework-for-Measuring-Nurses-Contributions-to-Care-Coordination

Limpahan, L.P., Baier, R.R., Gravenstein, S., Liebmann, O., & Gardner, R.L. (2013). Closing the loop: Best practices for cross-setting communication at ED discharge. *American Journal of Emergency Medicine, 31*(9), 1297-1301.

Mastal, M., & Palsbo, S. (2005). *Measuring the effectiveness of managed care for adults with disabilities.* Retrieved from http://www.chcs.org/resource/measuring-the-effectiveness-of-managed-care-for-adults-with-disabilities

McComb, S., & Simpson, V. (2014). The concept of shared mental models in healthcare collaboration. *Journal of Advanced Nursing, 70*(7), 1479-1488.

Naylor, M.D., & Ware, M.S. (2012, March 5). *Policy brief: The imperative for patient, family and population centered interprofessional approaches to care coordination and transitional care.* Philadelphia, PA: American Academy of Nursing.

Population Health Alliance. (2012). *Implementation and evaluation: A population health guide for primary care.* Washington, DC: Author.

Ryvicker, M., McDonald, M., Trachtenberg, M., Peng, T., Sridharan, S., & Feldman, P. (2013). Can the care transitions measure predict re-hospitalization risk or home health nursing use of home healthcare patients? *Journal for Healthcare Quality, 35*(5), 32-41.

Shaw, R.J., McDuffie, J.R., Hendrix, C.C., Edie, A., Lindsey-Davis, L., Nagi, A., ... Williams, J.W. (2014). Effects of nurse-managed protocols in the outpatient management of adults with chronic conditions: A systematic review and meta-analysis. *Annals of Internal Medicine, 161*(2), 113-122.

Smolowitz, J., Speakman, E., Wojnar, D., Whelan, E.M., Ulrich, S., Hayes, C., & Wood, L. (2015). Role of the registered nurse in primary health care: Meeting health care needs in the 21st century. *Nursing Outlook, 63*(2), 130-136.

Swan, B. A. (2012). A nurse learns first hand that you may fend for yourself after a hospital stay. *Health Affairs, 31*(11), 2579-2582.

Swan, B.A., & Haas, S. (2011). Health care reform: Current updates and future initiatives for ambulatory care nursing. *Nursing Economic$, 29*(6), 331-334.

Takach, M., & Yalowich, R. (2014). *Transforming the workforce to provide better chronic care: The role of nurse care managers in Rhode Island.* Retrieved from www.aarp.org/health/health-insurance/info-2014/role-of-nurse-care-managers-ri-AARP-ppi-health.html

Tomita, A., Lukens, E.P., & Herman, D.B. (2014). Assessing the role of family relations in reducing psychiatric re-hospitalization. *Psychiatric Rehabilitation Journal, 37*(1), 4-10.

Trehearne, B., Fishman, P., & Linn, E.H. (2014). Role of the nurse in chronic illness management: Making the medical home more effective. *Nursing Economic$, 32*(4), 178-185.

Weberg, D., & Weberg, K. (2014). Seven behaviors to advance teamwork. *Nursing Administration Quarterly, 38*(3), 230-237.

Wee, S., Loke, C., Liang, C., Ganesan, G., Wong, L., Cheah, J., & Med, M. (2014). Effectiveness of a national transitional care program in reducing acute care use. *The American Geriatrics Society, 62*(4), 747-753.

West, E., Holmes, J., Sidek, C., & Edwards, T. (2013). Intraprofessional collaboration through an unfolding case and the just culture model. *Journal of Nursing Education, 52*(8), 470-474.

Wiley, J.A., Rittenhouse, D.R., Shortell, S.M., Casalino, L.P., Ramsay, P.P., Bibi, S., & Alexander, J.A. (2015). Managing chronic illness: Physician practices increased the use of care management and medical home processes. *Health Affairs Online Journal, 34*(1), 780-786.

Young, J.M., Butow, P.N., Walsh, J., Durcinoska, I., Dobbins, T.A., Rodwell, L., & Solomon, M.J. (2013). Multicenter randomized trial of centralized nurse-led telephone-based care coordination to improve outcomes after surgical resection for colorectal cancer. *Journal of Clinical Oncology, 31*(28), 3585-3592.